ATHLETE'S FOOT

YET ANOTHER WAY OF DEALING WITH

ATHLETE'S FOOT

DR. J. SIMON

Contents

INTRODUCTION

Tinea pedis, often known as athlete's foot, is a common fungal infection that affects the skin on the feet, particularly between the toes. This disease is caused by several different types of fungi, including species of Trichophyton and Epidermophyton. Fungi thrive in an ideal environment, which is why athlete's foot is a common condition among people who play sports or partake in other activities that induce perspiration on the feet.

Vital Information

Infection linked to fungi:

Athlete's foot is the name given to a fungal infection that mostly affects the feet. Dermatophyte fungi, which prefer warm, humid environments to thrive, is the cause of it.

Normal Locations:

The illness can affect the tops, sides, and soles of the foot in addition to the area between the toes, which is where it frequently strikes. Periodically, it could spread to the toenails or other parts of the body.

Perilous Components

Athlete's foot is more common in those with weakened immune systems, tight or poorly ventilated shoes, sweaty feet, and bare feet in damp public areas like swimming pools or locker rooms.

Indications

The symptoms of athlete's foot can include burning, peeling, blistering, itching, and redness. The skin may get damaged or break in severe cases.

Easily Transferable Features:

Contact with infected people or contaminated surfaces, such as public restroom floors or towels, can result in the transmission of athlete's foot.

Preventive:

Wearing breathable shoes and moisture-wicking socks, avoiding going barefoot in public areas, and keeping clean, dry feet are some preventive measures. Antifungal powders and lotions are another.

Therapy:

The common treatment for athlete's foot is antifungal medication. These are either prescribed by a medical professional or available over-the-counter. For a satisfying result, it is imperative that you maintain good foot hygiene and follow recommended treatment methods.

Athlete's foot can occur repeatedly or chronically, even though it is usually mild and manageable. Maintaining proper hygiene, identifying symptoms early, and starting therapy on time all contribute to effective management. For an accurate diagnosis and recommended course of treatment, individuals with severe or ongoing instances should speak with a physician.

CHAPTER ONE

The fungi responsible for athlete's foot are dermatophytes, a type of fungal that prefers warm, humid environments. Swimming pools, public showers, and locker rooms are high-humidity areas where athlete's foot fungus is common. Some people are more susceptible to athlete's foot than others, and it can develop for a variety of reasons. Risk factors and causes include the following:

infection linked to fungi:

The etiology of athlete's foot is dermatophyte fungi, specifically Trichophyton and

Epidermophyton species. Certain fungi prefer warm, humid conditions, which makes the feet the ideal spot for them to grow.

Conditions: Warm and Wet:

Athlete's foot is caused by fungi that thrive in warm, humid environments. Accessing communal areas such as saunas, swimming pools, and locker rooms barefoot increases the risk of exposure.

Damp feet

Under the medical term hyperhidrosis, excessive perspiration can create a moist environment in shoes that is ideal for the growth of fungi. In those with sweaty feet, athlete's foot is more common.

Wearing Boots That Are Too Tight or Not Enough Air Vent:

The retention of heat and moisture in shoes that don't allow for adequate ventilation can promote the growth of fungus. Tight shoes can also irritate and rub against the skin, which promotes the growth of fungus.

In public spaces, walking barefoot:

Shower stalls, gym floors, and changing rooms are among the public spaces where direct contact with infected surfaces can result in the transmission of an athlete's foot infection.

Trading Specific Items:

If you share shoes, socks, or towels with someone who has the fungal sickness, your chances of getting it could increase. Fungal growth is a possibility due to their ability to dwell on objects and surfaces.

Decreased Immune Reaction

Fungal infections, including athlete's foot, may be more common in people whose immune systems have been weakened by diseases, medications, or treatments like chemotherapy.

The Presence of Molecules:

There may be a genetic predisposition for some persons to develop athlete's foot or to be susceptible to fungal infections.

Years old

Athletes and adults are more likely to have athlete's foot. Due to their decreased time spent in public settings, children are less prone to suffer from this sickness.

Earlier Skin Conditions:

Fungal infections are more common in those with pre-existing skin conditions such as psoriasis or eczema because they have compromised skin barriers.

Diabetic:

Diabetes increases the risk of fungal infections, including athlete's foot, because of compromised immune systems and impaired circulation.

To avoid athlete's foot, it's critical to understand these causes and contributing variables. Wearing breathable shoes, avoiding going barefoot in public areas, and maintaining good foot hygiene can all significantly reduce the risk of this fungal illness.

Symptoms

Usually affecting the feet, tinea pedis, the fungus that causes athlete's foot, takes hold. Various symptoms may arise from it, varying in possible intensity. Athlete's foot commonly manifests as the following:

It hurts

Persistent itching, especially between the toes, is a common symptom of athlete's foot. The itching can range in intensity from mild to severe and can be exacerbated by moisture and heat.

Both red and swollen:

Redness and swelling may appear on the affected skin. If left untreated, athlete's foot can also affect the tops and sides of the feet in addition to the area between the toes and the soles.

A Dim Sentiment:

A lot of persons with athlete's foot on their affected area experience burning or stinging sensations. After you take off your shoes and socks, this stiffness could become more noticeable.

Eczema with Peeling Skin:

Peeling or flaking skin is a common side effect of athlete's foot. Along with the space between the toes, this may also affect the sides and soles of the foot.

Scratches or breaks:

Small blisters or skin fissures may result from athlete's foot in more severe cases. Pain may result from these holes, which may increase the risk of further bacterial infections.

Bad Odor:

Fungus-related illnesses can occasionally produce an offensive odor, like athlete's foot. This smell is often the result of the interaction between the skin's fungi and bacteria.

Type: Dry Skin

Dry, scaly skin might be an indication of athlete's foot symptoms. Pain and irritability could get worse as a result.

Toenail Changes:

Onychomycosis, a fungal nail infection, is occasionally the outcome of athlete's foot. Toenail brittleness, thickening, or discolouration are possible.

Remember that athlete's foot can spread to other parts of the body, such as the hands and groin, if it is not treated quickly. In case you suspect athlete's foot or find your symptoms troublesome, it is advisable to consult a physician. Antifungal medications available over-the-counter and good foot hygiene are often beneficial in the treatment of athlete's foot.

Identification and Evaluation of the Medical

In order to diagnose athlete's foot, a medical professional will often do an examination. A diagnosis is made based on the following procedures and considerations:

Medical Evaluation:

An expert in medicine will do a clinical examination of the affected areas, paying particular attention to the feet. Together with other skin anomalies, they'll be watching for telltale signs and symptoms including peeling, redness, itching, and inflammation.

Patient's medical history:

The healthcare practitioner will inquire about the patient's past medical history, as well as any history of fungal infections, exposure to potential infection sources (such as shared areas like swimming pools or gym showers), and the duration and progression of the patient's symptoms.

Visual Inspection

Looking at the affected skin, typical patterns associated with athlete's foot can be seen, such as involvement of the sides, soles, and spaces between the toes. Blisters, fissures, or scaling may also be visible in progress.

In rare circumstances, the skin that is affected may be examined using UV radiation from a Wood's lamp. Certain fungus illnesses may glow when exposed to UV light, which could aid in diagnosis.

Lab Exams:

While not generally necessary, laboratory testing might be ordered by healthcare experts to confirm the diagnosis. Skin scrapings from the affected area may need to be taken for microscopic investigation or fungal culture in order to identify the exact type of fungus.

Separating This Situation from Others:

Similar to those of athlete's foot are the signs and symptoms of bacterial infections, psoriasis, and eczema. A physician may need to differentiate between different conditions in order to provide an accurate diagnosis.

It is imperative that those suffering with athlete's foot consult a physician in order to obtain a precise diagnosis and appropriate management. OTC antifungal medication treatment and self-diagnosis may not always be effective. This is especially true if there are complicating factors or if the infection is misdiagnosed.

Antifungal medications are often administered topically (to the skin) for more serious infections or taken orally once a diagnosis has been made. Keeping the feet clean and dry, avoiding situations that promote the growth of fungi such as wearing tight shoes or wet socks and practicing good foot hygiene are other effective ways to manage and prevent athlete's foot.

Therapy Techniques

For athlete's foot, antifungal medications and good foot hygiene are standard therapies. Typically, athlete's foot is treated using the following techniques:

Topical Antifungals:

Antifungal lotions, ointments, and sprays available over-the-counter (OTC) are often beneficial for mild instances of athlete's foot. A few examples of common active ingredients are clotrimazole, miconazole, terbinafine, and tolnaftate. You should apply these medications to the affected regions in accordance with the instructions on the product package.

Medications that require a prescription:

A medical expert may prescribe stronger topical antifungal medications for more severe or persistent instances of athlete's foot. They could be prescription-strength creams or oral antifungal medications.

Antifungal medications taken orally:

In case of a serious infection or damage to the toenails, prescription medications such as terbinafine or itraconazole could be suggested. Typically, doctors only give these oral medications for more serious illnesses.

Combination Therapy:

An oral and topical antifungal medication combination may be recommended by doctors for a more comprehensive course of therapy if the infection is severe or damages the nails.

Powders that are antifungal:

To keep the fungus at bay and the feet dry, apply antifungal sprays or powders inside shoes or directly on the feet. This could be an early warning system or part of the treatment plan.

Keeping Up Adequate Foot Cleaning

In order to prevent and treat athlete's foot, you must maintain clean feet. Every day washing, thorough drying, especially between the toes, and frequent sock changes are essential for maintaining healthy feet. Avoid wearing shoes that are too tight or have inadequate ventilation.

Avoid Reactive Substances:

Since irritants can worsen their condition, athletes should avoid them. Applying irritants to the affected areas, washing with harsh soaps, and wearing wet socks are all part of this.

Handling Moisture:

Dry feet are necessary when treating athlete's foot. Wearing socks that wick away moisture, choosing breathable shoes, and thoroughly drying the feet after washing are all necessary to achieve this.

Contaminated Items Separation:

Athlete's foot can spread easily, thus people should take precautions to avoid doing so. Towels, socks, and shoes should not be shared with other people. Instead, shoes and shower surfaces should be cleaned.

It is imperative that you follow the prescribed treatment plan consistently, even if symptoms go away before the suggested duration. People should see a healthcare provider if the infection worsens or shows no progress in order to have additional evaluation and adjustment of the treatment strategy.

CHAPTER TWO

Proactive Measures

The prevention of athlete's foot is crucial in halting its start and recurrence. Several useful techniques to prevent athlete's foot are as follows:

Keeping Up Adequate Foot Cleaning

Daily foot washing with soap and water should include cleaning in between your toes. A spotless foot is a must, therefore pay close attention to the spaces between your toes where moisture tends to gather.

Retain your dry feet:

A damp environment is the ideal one for fungi to grow. A completely dry foot is a must after taking a bath, going swimming, or engaging in any other water-related activity. When using a new towel, make sure the spaces between the toes are dry.

Picking Out Air-Cooling Shoes:

Wear shoes with mesh or leather uppers or other breathable materials to encourage airflow. Avoid wearing airtight, tight shoes as they cause moisture retention and encourage the formation of fungus.

Take Off Your Shoes:

To give each pair of shoes an opportunity to air out, rotate them after each wear. By doing this, you can prevent moisture buildup and lower your risk of developing fungal infections.

Moisture Wicking Socks Don Socks':

Wear socks made of materials that wick away moisture, such as wool or synthetic blends, to help keep your feet dry. Sock replacement is advisable, particularly if the socks become damp.

Avoid Wearing Only Your Soles in Public:

In public areas such as gym showers, locker rooms, and swimming pools, avoid wearing barefoot. A warm, moist environment is conducive to the growth of fungus, which opens up potential infection sites.

Spritz or powder antifungals:

Treat your feet and shoes with antifungal sprays or powders, especially if you are prone to fungal infections. The atmosphere for the growth of fungi may become less conducive as a result.

Maintain Trim Nails:

Keep your toe nails neat and manicured. A fungus that infects toenails can sometimes cause onychomycosis.

Keep Your Own Items to Yourself:

A person who may have a fungal infection should not share shoes, socks, towels, or other personal items. Exchanging items can help spread athlete's foot because it is an infectious condition.

Look Often at Your Feet:

Look for any signs of skin changes, redness, or irritation on your foot on a regular basis. In order to prevent the infection from spreading, prompt identification can help with immediate action.

Uphold Proper Hand Sanitization:

Remember to wash your hands properly after handling your feet or using an antifungal medicine. This can prevent the growth of fungus on other persons or in other parts of your body.

By adopting these preventive measures into your daily routine, you can reduce your risk of developing athlete's foot and maintain overall foot health. In case you have ongoing symptoms or suspect an infection, promptly seek medical attention for a diagnosis and treatment.

Lifestyle Adjustments and Foot Maintenance

Proper foot care and lifestyle changes can improve overall foot health and reduce the occurrence of athlete's foot in addition to specific preventive strategies. The ensuing recommendations are offered:

Choosing the Appropriate Footwear

Select footwear that has enough ventilation. Choose clothing items made of breathable fabrics, such as leather or mesh. A warm, wet environment that promotes the growth of fungi may be created by wearing shoes that are too tight or constricting.

Flip Your Shoes Around:

To let your shoes breathe, turn them around and don't wear the same pair every day. In addition to reducing moisture buildup, this allows shoes more time to dry entirely.

Frequently Check Your Feet:

Seek for any surprising changes, peeling, or redness on your feet often. An early diagnosis can prevent the spread of sickness and allow for prompt treatments.

Use caution when trimming toenails:

Toenails should be clipped straight across; avoid cutting them too short. Taking good care of your nails will protect you from cuts that can become infected with fungi.

Moisturize Dry Skin:

Dry or cracked skin needs to be moisturized just as much as keeping your feet dry is important. Use a mild moisturizer to prevent harsh dryness, particularly on the heels.

Avoid Wearing Only Your Soles in Public:

Take care when entering public areas like gyms, pools, and locker rooms barefoot. Cover your feet with flip-flops or shower shoes to protect them from any fungal infections.

Fully Dry Feet:

Check that your feet are completely dry after washing them, paying special attention to the spaces in between your toes. Wipe your feet dry with a clean towel, making sure to avoid leaving any damp areas that can attract fungus.

Ensure that your towels, socks, and bed linens are clean. Washing and replacing these things on a regular basis will help keep your feet clean and prevent fungus from growing.

Reduce Your Perspiration:

Wearing moisture-wicking socks and changing them during the day might be a good idea if your feet sweat a lot. The soles of your feet should be treated with antiperspirant to assist reduce excessive sweating.

In public areas, remember to practice proper foot hygiene.

Take extra care when using public showers and changing spaces by donning flip-flops or shower shoes. Being really hygienic means washing your feet thoroughly after being in public places.

Contemplate about powder for feet:

Your risk of fungal infections can be reduced by using antifungal foot powders or talcum powder to keep your feet dry.

Treat Illnesses That Last Long:

To address any underlying conditions, like diabetes, that may affect the health of your feet and reduce the risk of problems, work closely with your healthcare provider.

By incorporating these foot care practices and lifestyle modifications, you can maintain the health of your feet and reduce your risk of developing athlete's foot or other foot-related issues. Should you experience persistent symptoms or worry about the condition of your feet, consult a medical professional for advice and treatment.

Handling Consequences and Repeats

To treat the recurrence and consequences of athlete's foot, preventive measures, appropriate therapy, and ongoing foot care are require. Complications and recurrence can be managed with the help of these strategies:

Complete Programs for Therapy:

Be sure you take all oral or topical antifungal medications according to stated dosages. The chance of an infection persisting or reoccurring is higher when therapy ends early.

Observe precautionary measures:

Continue with the preventive measures, such as wearing shoes with plenty of ventilation, keeping your feet dry, and giving your feet proper attention. With these treatments, athlete's foot might not come back.

Routine inspections of the feet:

Regularly check your own feet for any early signs of athlete's foot or other foot issues. By acting early, complications can be prevented.

Avoid triggers at all costs.

Ascertain any possible triggers that may lead to a recurrence of athlete's foot and avoid them. This can include going barefoot, neglecting to take care of your feet, or venturing into public spaces without the proper footwear.

Consider the following maintenance therapy:

Medical doctors may recommend topical antifungal maintenance medication in select cases to try to prevent recurrence of athlete's foot. In order to control the infection, this means taking the medication regularly.

Manage the underlying circumstances.

Unmanaged medical conditions, such as immune system disorders or diabetes, may be the cause of recurrent fungal infections. Working together with your healthcare provider will help you manage these problems effectively.

Consult a Health Care Provider:

If, despite taking precautions, athlete's foot recurs, a thorough evaluation by a medical professional is necessary. They possess the ability to assess the underlying causes and offer appropriate adjustments to the therapeutic plan.

CHAPTER THREE

Address problems right away:

If problems arise, such recurring bacterial infections or toenail involvement, get medical help right away. To treat consequences, other treatments could be required, such as specialist care for fungal nail infections or antibiotics for bacterial infections.

Consider Shoe Cleaning:

To eliminate any potential fungus, regularly sanitize your shoes. You could do this by using antifungal powders or sprays inside the shoes.

Frequently flip your shoes to allow the air to escape and reduce the possibility of fungus growing. Avoid going about your entire day in the same shoes.

Have a Podiatrist Conversation:

If you often experience athlete's foot or problems with your toenails, consult a podiatrist or other foot specialist. Personalized treatment and counseling can be provided in accordance with your unique needs.

Appropriate and prompt treatment is essential to prevent complications and reduce the likelihood of recurrence of athlete's foot. By including these precautions into your routine and seeking professional counsel when needed, you may be able to treat athlete's foot more effectively and maintain optimal foot health.

CONCLUSION

All things considered, athlete's foot is a common fungal disease that primarily affects the feet and is characterized by symptoms of peeling, redness, and itching. If left untreated, athlete's foot can become persistent and have implications even though it is generally not a serious condition. Managing athlete's foot requires a mix of intensive therapy, early detection, and ongoing foot care.

By implementing preventive measures, such as choosing appropriate footwear, keeping feet clean, and avoiding potential infection sources, the frequency of athlete's foot can be considerably reduced. The treatment of contributing factors such excessive dampness, early symptom detection, and frequent foot exams are all part of preventive care.

For the fungus to be eradicated, athlete's foot must be treated as soon as symptoms arise. Prompt foot hygiene and topical and oral antifungal medications are essential for an effective course of treatment. Complete adherence to the recommended medication regimen is essential to prevent complications and relapses.

One way to prevent recurrences is to identify potential triggers and steer clear of them, consider maintenance therapy under the guidance of a qualified practitioner, and seek comprehensive examinations from medical professionals. Treatment of underlying medical conditions and prompt medical attention for any difficulties, such as bacterial infections or involvement of the toenail, are crucial parts of complete care.

Some examples of good foot care techniques that can enhance your overall foot health and reduce your risk of acquiring athlete's foot include checking your feet on a regular basis, trimming your toenails, and wearing dry shoes. Consulting with medical professionals that specialize in podiatry can provide tailored advice and targeted therapy when needed.

Athlete's foot can ultimately be treated if the right combination of foot care, medication, and prevention is used. By incorporating these precautions into daily activities and exercising caution, people can reduce the detrimental effects of athlete's foot on their overall health and enjoy comfortable, healthy feet.

THE END